Running Kit for Beginners

Practical Steps to Start Running

Maya Loan – Paolo Menescardi

Table of Contents

Introduction

Hello and thank you for taking the time to check out and read this book!

Running is something that can change your life. For some, it's a therapeutic habit. For others, it's a way to get in shape. For some, it is actually a way to help you maintain a sound mind and a sound body. Running does a lot for a person, and it can definitely be a good thing to do.

However, many people shy away from running. The stress of it all, the problems associated with it, the ability to not spend time with it, all of these are hurdles that many put forward that stop you from running.

Let's face it, if we went around and asked people why they don't run or exercise, they would say, "I don't have the time" or "I don't feel like I can ever be good at running anyways." In reality, everyone can be good at it, but it does take mastering a good pace, starting from the bottom, and working from there.

Even just running at an even pace for about 15 minutes will suffice when you're starting out, and from there you can evolve into not just a beginner runner, but someone who can hold their ground in a race. Starting with about thirty minutes of running and going from there will do you a whole lot of good. In truth, it isn't hard to start running, and this book will give you a comprehensive guide to running and how to get into it.

This book will take you from the person that you are, someone who doesn't run, and morph you into the person that you've wanted to be, which is a runner. It won't take long, and in truth, once you have your mind set on it, it'll make things even better.

Running is a skill, and it does take time to master, but with this book, you'll be able to master the art of running and become a runner yourself.

I used to have a disdain for running. Never thought I could get into it. However, after a while I started to learn more about running, and from there, I grew to love the sport. I started to realize that I could become a way better runner, and in truth, I started to do so. I want everyone to learn how to run adequately, and in truth, once you get started, you won't want to stop.

Chapter 1: starting on Your Running Journey

The biggest hurdle really isn't running, but rather it's the decision to run. Most people think that running is something boring, something that isn't a fun endeavor, but that's far from the truth. Running is a great activity, but you need to know how to start before you can get anywhere with it. This book will go over how to get started on your journey to being the best runner

Getting the Urge to Start

Now, the first hurdle you will go over, and I'm sure it won't be easy for you but you'll have to bear with it in order to get anywhere with running, is the desire to start.

Naturally, when you first start running your mind will think of everything that it can do besides run. You will try to make excuses, get away from it, and in general, you won't want to do it subconsciously. Sure, you want to, but you should make sure that you dedicate time to this. Schedules will be discussed in the next chapter, but you need to have the desire to do it.

You want to have a goal in mind as well. Goals are so important when you're starting on this journey. For one, if you don't have a goal at all fitness-wise, you won't get anywhere. Many people struggle with fitness activities because most of the time they're working aimlessly with no goal. Many times, the reasons why people quit the gym, quit running, or anything of the sort, are because they don't have any drive in their body to do this. To rectify that, you need to have a goal before you go.

This goal can be as simple as you want to lose five pounds, or you want to run for longer than an hour without running out of breath, or you're training for a running activity such as a 5K or something of the sort. Whatever it may be, it's on you. Choose a goal that won't be problematic of jarring from what you want to have in life. In general, make it a realistic goal, something that won't be super hard for you to maintain, but is enough of a challenge that you're working to make it. You shouldn't try to make the goal immediately be running a marathon, although you can after a while. With running, it does take some effort to really get to where you want to go with it, which is why it's important that you keep your goal within your head and work towards it when you can.

Dress Correct

A common thing many people who start out with running suffer from is they try to get so many things prepared for running, when in essence it requires a few things. You need to have the appropriate clothing for running, and this section will go over what you need to do, the initial clothing you should get, and some of the best choices.

Your biggest choice is shoes. Shoes can make or break a runner. I know this, because in the past I've bought shoes that were good for a couple of weeks, but then I started to get shin splints from this. If you buy the wrong type of shoes, you'll run into problems. For many who start out, they tend to get the generic brands of shoes when they're starting out. While that might work for a couple of weeks, if you're serious about this, you've got to get shoes that are fitting for you.

For those who want something that supports shins, typically Asics are good. New balance is good for those who have wide feet. The Vibrams shoes are good in some cases, but they've been known to cause shin and knee problems in some. The best thing to do is to go to a running store and ask them to personally help you find the right shoe. Do take them for a small test drive around the store, and if they feel comfy, get them. If you have arches that are low, I suggest getting Dr. Scholl's or an orthotic if you're willing to pay the price. They can significantly help your arches and help to prevent shin splints or any other problems.

For clothing, you want to get what's right for you. For women, typically the dry-fit tops, running tanks, and sports bras are good for you upper body. With a sports bra, get one that supports you. Nike bras and tops are pretty good, and usually trying them on and feeling the support of them is a good thing to start with. When it comes to bottoms, you have many choices. You can do running leggings, which are great for when they're cold. They're really comfy and they fit well. Shorts are also good; just get the typical running shorts or the dry fit ones, because they feel nice. Spandex is also nice to run in as well, but be wary of this, because often people buy them too tight, and it can be uncomfortable to start.

For guys, tanks and running shirts are good. For the bottoms, running shorts, compression shorts, or spandex are great. You can also get running socks too if you want

I would say if you're pressed for money to get some old shirts and some shorts from the store to start. They might not be the comfiest, but they work well for what you need. Also, do keep in mind that it might be cold when you run, so getting a sweatshirt or a hoodie can help. Long-sleeve tops also do the trick as well.

Finally, there are water bottles. In general, you want something thin. Typically, people like to run with water bottles in their hands, or if you are on a track, you can leave it on the track. A big one might be good in some cases, but it can be bulky to carry, so I advise leaving the bigger water bottles at home and get something small and efficient. Don't get plastic bottles and refill them. For one, it's not good for you, so you shouldn't do that. Plus, it can get crinkly and gross fast.

Medical Visit

For some, the medical visit is another very important step. Medical visits are completely necessary for some people, since often they might not know if they have a condition or not. You should go to the doctor to get everything checked out. Ideally, you should be fit for running small distances, but if you have heart or breathing problems, it's advisable to go see your doctor.

They can also let you know how much you can do. For some people, they might have to start off with very gradual speeds, working up to the level that they can be at to run adequately. Whatever the case, you should go anyways because it's important to let your doctor know what's going on, how things are faring, and other elements too.

If you do have a medical condition that bars you from running long distances, do take this in mind. With every physical activity, you shouldn't overexert yourself. It's also good to make sure that you aren't prone to shin or knee injuries, because typically that's where the problems lie. If you have arches that are low as well, you can get orthotics from your doctor too if you're willing to pay for them. It's important to do this step, because it is a preliminary step that will help you.

Location

Location is a very important element to running. This section will go over the types of places to run, the pros of them, and the cons of them.

The first is running outside around your neighborhood. This is a good start, and it can help lead to something else. With this, you should make sure your neighborhood is safe to run in, and also take a look at the pathways. Sidewalks can be hard on some shins, so do keep that in mind when you are choosing a location.

There are also parks. This is one of the best places to go, because parks have a myriad of pathways most of the time, and you can then run around on these pathways. Plus, there are more grass and dirt paths, and you'll be able to make it easier on your shins and your body ultimately if you do this.

Then there are indoor tracks. Some gyms and fitness clubs have them, and you can use those in order to run and get your fitness on. These are good for starting out, and you can track how far you've run as well. Typically, indoor tracks are about 40 meters, and the outdoor are about the same as well, but they do vary. These are the best if you have one in your area that is open to the general public.

In general, find a path that works for you. If your area is super hilly, it might to be a good fit for you. For some, hills can be trying on the body, and when starting out it might set you up for losses. A place that has even terrain, or as even as you can get, is what will work best, and you can gradually go up from there to a course that is harder over time.

Diet

When you're running, your body will need the correct fuel to work. For many when they're first starting out, they don't realize that the food they're eating is hurting them. Many of us live on a high-sugar and high-carb diet, which is where the problems come in.

Sugar is necessary, but if you're eating too much processed sugar, it's not going to end well for you. With running, if you eat a bunch of sugar before you run, your body is as good as screwed. Your body will had bad fuel in its arsenal when you run, and over time it'll start to tire out. You should instead have natural sugars, but don't be afraid to have other foods as well.

When it comes to carbs, get rid of the simple ones, and instead get the complex carbs. Potatoes, lentils, beans, and other such foods have carbs in them, but they're good for you, and they can help your body.

For protein, you will want to have a lot of it. Meat, poultry, fish, some veggies, and other such foods are the way to go. Have this, since it will give your body fuel to work before you start to run around.

When it comes to when to eat, the answer is simple. Ideally, you should eat about an hour before you run. That way, your food has enough time to digest. If you can, eat only a little bit beforehand. You don't want to go into it with no food at all though. If you do that, you're setting yourself up for failure because your body won't have anything, and soon it'll be running on empty over time. You should instead, eat something light, but also full of vitamins and minerals.

When you're getting into the spirit of running, you should eat a rainbow of fruits and veggies. You're losing a lot of the vitamins you would typically have, since many vitamins are fat-soluble, and many are water-soluble, which means either way you're getting rid of some of the elements that you typically need. With that in mind, it's important to note that you should have at least some sort of supplements each day. It doesn't have to be a lot, but it can be enough to help you get along. I know when I'm running I do make sure to take all the supplements I'll need, or eat an array of vegetables. A multivitamin will typically hit all the right points.

For meals, you should eat before, and within the hour after you run. The reason for this is that if you don't eat after you run, your body will go into survival mode, and soon the fat won't leave your body. This is not a good thing to have happen, so it's important that you do eat. You should keep in mind your calories, but do also make sure you take into account your activity level as well, because the higher the activity level, the more calories you'll need over time.

These are the preliminary steps you must take when you're getting ready to run. It's important you know these, because making sure that you do them will make it a lot easier on you as well.

Chapter 2: The Importance of Schedules

Now beforehand, we did discuss a bit about schedules, but this chapter will go over the importance of them. A schedule can make or break your running regimen, and often, if you do run outside of your schedule, you won't have a lot of success with it. With this chapter, you'll learn some of the important reasons you run on a schedule, and why it's important.

The first is you'll keep at it if you have a schedule. I know people will time and time again say that they will go run, but then they never make an effort to do so. That's because they don't keep a schedule on hand. It's a rule of thumb that if you don't maintain a schedule to run, you won't do it. There will be other factors that "conveniently" come in. I know this, because when I first started I didn't really pay mind to it, but over time I did realize that a schedule is essential.

It also keeps you motivated. Often, if you don't have a schedule there, you won't be motivated to continue. This happens a lot, because humans typically need some incentive to do things, and it can be hard to really keep at it over time. For many of us, we do need to keep ourselves going and we need reassurance of what we're doing. A set schedule and strict following to it will help you with this.

It also will help you get more done. When we don't have a schedule set up in life, we don't really get what we need completed. The same goes for running. A schedule of when you'll run, what you'll do, where you'll go, and other such things, will help you significantly. If you don't have one, it makes the struggle all the more harder, and it can be a nightmare when getting stuff done. If you don't have a schedule as well, sometimes little problems will creep in, taking your attention off the running and back onto the problem at hand instead of doing something else.

With running, it's also important to keep in mind that a schedule will help you go further. Think about it, you pick a good time to do this, and you can extend it further when you're ready. Right now we'll only be going for up to 30 minutes, but once you're past the entry level, you'll want to do more typically. You might want to go for an hour run. If you don't have that set into your day, you won't have a chance to do it. Stop selling yourself short, and start to put this in, because it will allow you to improve over time as well.

Also, there is another part of this that many people don't realize can be problematic for people. That is the factor of eating. Many times, if you don't have a schedule, you'll go running at the worst possible times for you. Many people like to get their runs done first thing in the morning, and if for some reason they decide to not follow their schedule and do it at night, it could mix you up because of how much food you have within you. If your body isn't used to running with food inside of it, you shouldn't run with food inside to the point where it might hurt. It can cause cramping and other issues. Yes, having some sustenance before you go is essential because it gives you fuel to go, but if you had a big dinner and then go running, if you're not used to it the workout might ruin you and make you sick. Without a schedule, you might end up doing that, and after a few times, it can be really painful. You should run when you feel comfortable, and when you think it's right.

Now some can run on a full stomach. Everyone is different, and often, you have to figure out what works for you. I can't run on a full stomach, but I know someone who runs well in that manner. That person might do best working out after dinner, whereas with me I have to do it first thing or else I can get sick. In general, you will need to figure out what is right for you, find the schedule that works, and keep to it because if you don't, it can cause trouble for you later on.

For many people, scheduling can make or break your ability to keep at it, so it's important that you do keep these in mind when you are formulating your schedule. The next chapter will go over how to adequately do that to the point where you're getting the best results possible.

Chapter 3: The best schedule for running

The schedule for running that you want to have can be different in many cases. Everyone is a bit different, so you will want to make sure that you have something set up so that you're able to get somewhere with it. This chapter will go over the steps necessary to help you make the best schedule you can.

The first step is to first of all figure out the best time for you to go running. Like I said in the previous chapter, everyone is different. Some of us can take running right after we eat, or a little bit after we eat, but then there are others who can't have much when we run. For those who can run after you eat, you can do it at night. It's also cooler by then, so if you're not a fan of the heat, you'll be able to have a nice run.

For those who like to run on an empty or nearly empty stomach, first thing in the morning is what will work for you. It's also a good way to get into the groove before work. You might have to wake up a little bit early to do that, but it's worth it when your physical health is taken care of.

For those who don't want to run first thing in the morning or at night; then before dinner is another option. It's a bit busier at that time since everyone is at the park, the track, or they might be out and about getting home, but if it's comfortable for you, then do that.

At the end of it all, being comfortable is the end goal you want to have. It really do make it easier on you and you'll be motivated to do it if you do it within a time period that best fits your body.

Now that you have a time period during the day, it's time to focus on the scheduling blocks for running. In general, for starting you will want to do about 15 minutes planned out just for running. When you're going from the start, from step zero, up to entry-level runner, you won't have to spend much time at first actually running. You're going to need to build it up. I know people who start to wheeze after a minute of running. It happens, you just have to build yourself up from there. So when you start, expect about 15 minutes of your time to be spent with this activity, and then work it up from there.

For the first three minutes, you'll stretch. You might take a couple minutes longer, but if it can be done within the three minutes, do that. You can then start your clock, and then start to run.

With running, do it until you start to feel like you can't do it anymore. It might be a minute or it might be three minutes. Take a second to catch your breath, and then do it again. You can then end off with a bit of stretching if you desire.

When you first start, you'll walk a lot, but for the first day start with as far as you can and then increase it. Try to go up by about 15 seconds each time. It might be hard, but once you see you can do it, you'll feel better.

With that in mind, you are going to run into the point where you might have to extend you time. Eventually, you'll need about 40 minutes for a 30 minute run, sometimes a little bit less depending on how long you stretch or not. In general, have about 5 minutes dedicated to stretching as a good rule of thumb. You'll be able to limber up, and it'll help so you don't pull a muscle.

When you feel like you want to increase your time, you certainly can. Ideally, increase it within minute increments once you hit the thirty-minute mark. For some people, it might be a bit much, but do what best fits you. That's what you should be focused on, and that's what will help.

Doing what fits you is the goal for this, and having a schedule that best reflects it will help. You should block out the time you'll use for running, and then set up an alarm. With the alarm, you'll be able to calculate when you've got to go out and run. If you have to change into your workout clothes after dinner or after work, set up a reminder for that as well. If you have a reminder to do it, there is a much stronger chance that you will do it and get the job done.

With running, you should do it at your own pace. Don't be afraid to take a little bit more time than necessary. If you can leave about five minutes of leeway into your schedule in care if you do take your time a bit more, that can always help. You should do that especially if it's first thing in the morning, because all too often people are running around, and it can be a bit hard to keep yourself going and maintaining a schedule, so do make sure if you need to add the leeway, do so.

The next thing to do once you have the schedule is to test run it. Do a couple days at that schedule and see if it works. Now, if it works, keep at it and just work on extending the time at that point. If you feel like it's not working for you or the time isn't good for you, then it's best if you do choose a better time for yourself. Do work with what is best for you, what will help you get the most results from this, and do make sure that you take all of these into consideration when you run.

Having the best schedule that you can will, also, help you improve your ability to run. Doing it what your own pace, on your own terms, and with your determination in mind will allow you to have a better experience as well. Remember, you're doing this for you, so the schedule should reflect on what you want it to be, and over time, you'll be able to increase the pace and tempo, and you can also increase the time to further better yourself as well.

Chapter 4: Technological Support for Running

Now, with running, sometimes there is some technological support you can use. There are some apps you should have for distance, time, or even your own personal music if you want to use that. This chapter will go over the best running apps that will help you out.

Music Players

If you don't already have songs programmed onto your phone, having some music apps can help. IHeartradio, Spotify, and Pandora are great choices for this. The reason for these is because they can give you some music to choose from, and if you need something immediately, there is always YouTube to help. If you want to, you can also preload music and podcasts onto your phone before you start running to make it even better.

Runkeeper

This is a running app that many runners use. It will use the GPs to help you track how far you've ran, and you can use it for other distance activities as well. You can use it for pace, distance, your exercise time, and other metrics as well. You can also use it to help tag pictures as well. You can even use it to help with running routes too, and it will help you measure how fast you've gotten and your workout history too.

5K Runner

If your ultimate goal is to run a 5K, this is for you. For some running apps, it can be hard to start with them. However, this app is actually geared towards helping you get yourself ready for a 5K in about eight weeks. With this, you'll be able to run the 3.1 miles at the end of it, which is a good goal for some people. This comes with an audio coach that will help you stay motivated and even tell you what to do. It will help with tracking the pace, tell you how far you've gone, your heart rate, and even how many calories you're burning and if you're improving. There are also in inspirational quotes and other badges to help with the motivation. This is a great start for those branching out, and it can help you get the best results possible.

Zombies Run

With the obsessive appeal of zombies these days, you might be looking at the name and getting a chuckle. But let's face it, we've all seen zombie movies, or maybe played a video game or watched zombie TV shows, but what if you programmed it for real life? What if you used zombies to help you get running? Well, this is a good one if you want to make your running an exhilarating experience. In this, you will run, and literally run in this case, and you will try to get supplies, help people, and other such things, all while being chased by zombies. It's actually a very gripping app and even comes with sound effects. If you lower your pace, the zombies get closer, so you can sue this to help increase your pace while training.

MapMyRun

This is one of the most popular apps that are present on the app store, and it's a great running app for those with iPhones. It's built to work with an iPhone, and it even works with the other fitness devices you might have as well. It tells you of your pace, the route you're taking, the calories, and even other vital fitness stats that might be interesting. You can even equip your running shoes to the app and with it, you can monitor when you've got to get a new pair, which is what you should do after 300 miles. It's one of the best and simplest apps, and with the social media reach it has, it can be a great one for those starting out.

Endomondo

If you're looking for a running app that allows you to set a distance, calorie goal, or time with a coach that actually helps you, then this is the way to go. With this, you'll be able to use an interface that will allow you to work with this and help you get to your goals. You can connect it to the Apple health app and other fitness devices if you want to help track your workout data. The best thing about this app is that you can also connect with others via social media, and it can be used to challenge people, help give pep talks, and even share workouts with others. This is a great app for literally any distance you want, so whether you're entraining for a marathon, which might be your ultimate goal, or if you're just working to run for 30 minutes, this is the way to go.

Fitbit

The Fitbit is an interesting system that can be used to help you track overall health stats. It also tells you how many steps you take each day.

Now, with the steps, it is nice to know that, but that's not what you're going for with this. It's a good app for some to track how far you can walk, but you can use it for distance, and even to track vitals in people. For some, this is a good app to have in general to help with your overall health, and it's something that will certainly assist you in really learning about where to go and what sort of measures to take. A Fitbit is a bit pricy, but it's a good technological support if you're looking for one.

Media Player

Now, these apps can be downloaded right onto a smartphone, but sometimes, you might just want some music and a clock. Ideally, you should minimally have some type of media player, and a clock to help keep you going and knowing what time it is. For many people, a smartphone does the trick, but if you don't feel like bringing your phone with you, a simple iPod touch, or even an MP3 player is the way to go. Music is a great support that will keep you motivated when you run. I know that when I'm having a rough run, the right song can pop up and I'll be able to get through it, so having the support of media and listening to it can really make your runs all the more better as well.

Adidas Train and Run

Now the train and run is an expert fitness app that actually turns your phone into a personal trainer. This is good for those who love to slack or have trouble really getting started and going through with this. All too often, it can be hard to keep to it, but if you're looking to really get in shape and have a good workout, this is for you.

The app is great for beginners and advanced people alike, because it actually will give you real-time visual and audio feedback, which will allow you to have better training and allow you to stay active regardless. You'll be able to see the history of your workouts and how you're doing, the curves of your heart rate, and even maps of your previous routes. This will also give you other insights to allow you to have a great idea of where to go and how to increase the productivity of your workout.

This app is also good with the Fitsmart as well, which is an app that allows you to track everyday activities and show you the effort you're making to achieve a goal. It's also a great app that is completely free, so you're getting all of these benefits without too much of a problem with the price tag, that's for sure.

Rock My Run

Now, let's say that you love to run, and you have a set of songs in your arsenal. But let's say that you don't really like going through some of the songs that seem slow when you're running, and you're not feeling inspired with it. Well, research has proven that if you listen to lively and upbeat types of music, you can improve your performance and have a great impact on your time. It really can be the difference between really getting the workout you want, and not having the push to go forward.

This app does just that, in that it will give you great workout music so you'll have the energy needed to keep going while you run. It's got some great playlists and it will help give you a song with a high beats per minute to give you a great workout experience. You can even have the app integrate the rhythm of the songs and the tempo of songs to match the steps you make. It will help you get an even more in-depth workout, and it works with you will be able to use it together with other apps to help you really get the best workout experience that you can, and to really help you take that step forward.

Bluetooth Headphones

Now, normally you can start off with any old headphones, but there is something great about Bluetooth headsets. For starters, they are cheap these days. You've probably seen then go online for about 20 bucks, and let me tell you, that twenty bucks will be twenty well spent. They

Be simple, but so effective. They can be controlled by a push of a button, so if you want to skip a song you can. You won't have to hold onto your phone with this headset. The life of these is long as well. You won't have to replace them every so often like normal earbuds, and the sound quality is great. A Bluetooth headset is a great item to have in general to listen to music, and with how cheap they are these days, they're an item worth mentioning.

Technological support is integral to running for many people, especially in this Internet age. You should have the right apps to help you, and this chapter shows you just what types of apps are out there, and what can be used to further assist you.

Chapter 5: Training Schemes to Help You Become a Better Runner

Now, there are a few training regimens that you can do, and there are some great training activities that you can use to help you become the best runner that you can be. This chapter will go over a few of the amazing training activities that you can use to help you get the most you can.

The start

For starting, the best way to get yourself moving is to take your first step, bend the leg slightly, then put your foot down. Start going heel toe, and don't put too much stress on your body. You should keep your arms naturally at the side, and don't try to tense them up, because then that cramps up an area between your shoulder and neck, which is really painful. Do that, and just run on the flat surface for as long as you can. You should go until you feel like you can't go anymore. For some, this might be a minute. For others, this might be five minutes. When you're doing this, work up from there. Take it slow, and start to work on your form too. Ideally, you should be putting all of your attention on your form, and at the end of it, do track the time and distance. Try to go as long as you can, and then over time, you can increase the time from there.

An Incline

If you're feeling adventurous, or if you're craving a challenge, one of the best ways to get a challenge while running is an incline. I wouldn't suggest starting off with more than one incline, but choose an incline that is small but enough to pose a bit of a challenge. Go up it, keeping the pace that you normally go. You might struggle with this initially, but that's okay. Everyone has a bit of a struggle with hills at times, but you will want to start off slow and then go faster from there. Start with that one incline, and then do it once a session to help you train yourself.

Hill Runs

Okay, so let's say you've mastered your form, you feel a bit better about inclines, and you're ready to take on a hill. Find a place with a hill that is challenging enough for you, and start with it.

To start, go up it once. Push yourself as you go up it, and then relax on the decline. With all of these, you should try to push the incline as much as possible, and then go very slow on the decline. The reason for this is that you will naturally start to move faster because of how the decline is and gravity when you're going down. If you go at the same pace you do going up, you won't really get the best benefits that you can from it. Work the incline, and then relax on the decline.

At first, you might feel winded after the first hill, which is okay. Hill runs are hard, that's for sure. They aren't something you can easily do because often, they do take a bit of practice before it becomes easier for you. With that in mind though, work on the one hill till it gets easy enough where it's not as much of a struggle going up. After that, you can add another and work from there.

This is a great workout if you're looking to have defined calves. If you're looking for full leg definition, this is also good too. You can eventually graduate up to the point where you dedicate an entire training session to hills. What that means is you will go up and down the hills, pushing the incline then relaxing the decline, and do that for the allotted time. Try to see as many hills as you can get with this. It is a workout, that's for sure, but it's a fun workout that will really help you build yourself up. You shouldn't do this until you get to the entry-level point, so don't push yourself too hard at first.

Indian Run (intervals)

This is another very popular training technique for those who are working to get from beginner level to entry level and are closer to the entry level. If you're at step 0, stay with just trying to increase your time before you do any of these. If you feel you're ready for the challenge, you can do this form of training to assist you.

With this, you will run at a normal pace for about two minutes, and then run super fast one minute. This might seem like a simple routine, but do this multiple times. If you're able to run for about 20 minutes, you will do this multiple times, and in truth, it is tiring. You can combine this with hills if you're really adventurous, but in truth, if you start off with just doing it slower for a couple minutes, then faster for a short period of time, it does work. You can change up the times if doing it for a minute is too long, such as running at a normal pace for a minute and then going fast for about 30 seconds. This is a fun interval training, and if you're looking for a challenge, doing this alone will help you.

Track Running

For some people, running on tracks can help keep them focused. Track running can get a bit boring, but a good way to push yourself, is to see how many laps you can get done in a certain period of time. For example, you can choose to go for about 15 minutes, and from there, you see how many laps you can get done. This is a fun little challenge, and if you work on trying to go a bit faster than you did the last time, you will get better. You do need to take some time to perfect it, but over time, if you start to use the track, you will definitely have a much better experience.

These various training techniques will help you run better. In truth, these sessions can be used for a small period of time, or for a larger period of time, and it can be used to great results. In truth, it might take a bit of getting used to, and it can be something that does become a bit hard at first, but over time, you will be able to improve your running speeds and distances, and your times can become better as well. You've just got to train, and these different schemes can help you do so.

Chapter 6: The Benefits of Running

Now, there are a lot of benefits to running that are of note. For some people, they don't realize just what it can do. This chapter will go over some of the major benefits of running, and why running is one of the best activities to start with.

Lose Weight Fast

For many people, they start running because they want to lose weight. It's a good activity to get into, because running burns a lot of calories. In a run, you can burn about 300 calories at a normal pace, sometimes even more. You can also build up muscle with this, which is something that many people want to have but they don't. Muscle burns a lot more tan fat, so you'll be losing more weight if you add running to this.

A good diet does help you lose weight, but running will further help with this, and it does give you muscle. It will allow you to really have a much better time, and in general, it can be something that you can use to help with the trouble areas. You can help get rid of some of the fat on your body with this, and it does work.

Lowers Blood Pressure

High blood pressure can lead to many things you don't want to have, such as strokes, heart disease, and other afflictions. High blood pressure is something older individuals suffer from, and while diet is a very crucial element to this, running does lower it. If you run, it helps improve the cardiovascular system, which in turn will help make it more efficient. A more efficient cardiovascular system will help lower the blood pressure, and it can also help to loosen the plaque around your arteries if you have any. If you have high blood pressure, this can be a great thing for you.

Beat Heart Disease

Heart disease is the number one killer in America today. The diets we have, the lack of exercise we engage in, and all of these things are what attribute to cardiovascular issues. Heart disease can kill you, and if you're not careful it can creep up on you. Your cardiovascular system is something you should keep strong, and that's what running will do for you.

Your heart will pump blood faster, which in turn will move the blood around the body faster and more efficiency. This creates a stronger heart, and it will reduce the risk for a heart attack or a stroke. You'll be able to work out longer and you will be able to maintain a better heart rate as well. Don't let heart disease become a part of your life, and beat it with running so that you can lower your blood pressure greatly.

Improve Mood

We all go through bad moods. Moods can change drastically, and often, if we have a bad day, the last thing we think about doing is running. But, running releases endorphins in the body, which is a happy hormone that will make you feel better. In turn, you will feel happier, more relaxed, and it can help you have a better mood as well. Sometimes, the real cure for a bad day isn't sitting around eating ice cream, but rather It's going out for a little bit and doing something about it. Even if it is only for a couple of minutes, it can release enough endorphins in the body to make you feel better.

Relieves stress

Stress is another major problem we all suffer from. Stress can be really downing, and in truth, we do suffer from it many times just in our daily lives. If you have a job that can be trying on you, you'll need an activity to relieve it. With running, you can help make that stress wash away.

For one, you will be focused on what your body is doing and on the environment, and in truth it can help you to relieve the problems that you suffer from. It can help take away any frustrations that you have, and in turn you'll feel lighter. You'll be focused on what you're doing and not the zillions of other problems that you can suffer from. Instead of always worrying, take some time to run and relax, because the stress will only make you older and you won't feel as good.

Beat Depression

Depression is another major problem that people suffer from. If you do suffer from chronic depression, you might not feel like going out to run. But, running does relieve the effects of depression. The reason of that is because you're taking the attention off of what your body is doing, and instead you're putting it forward and out into the environment. It doesn't take much for you to do, and because of the endorphins, you will naturally feel happier and better as well.

Now, it might not permanently relieve the effects of it. But, if you feel like you're about to go crazy because of your depression, it can be a great way to help you feel better.

Have Better Sleep

If you're working out and running, naturally you'll feel tired. Your body will want to sleep, but not only that, you're taking your mind off other things when you start to sleep. Running can help you clear your mind, help to improve your sleeping schedule, and it can give you enough exercise to where you will sleep better. Studies have shown that with running, you will get better sleep. So you should do so, and if you can do it before bed, the results will be even better.

Confidence Booster

For many people, confidence is an issue and is hard to resolve. However, running gives you a chance to set goals for yourself. It doesn't have to be a huge goal; maybe just going a bit further than you did before. For many people, running does improve confidence, and with setting these goals and working on them, you will feel better and feel way more confident than you have felt before. Plus, it can tone up and improve your figure, so you might even feel better because of that.

Disease preventer

Yes, running does prevent disease. In women, running can help lower your chances for breast cancer. As said before, it does help with heart disease, and it will help to decrease the risk for stroke in people. For those who have early diabetes, high blood pressure, or even osteoporosis, it can help to improve all of these, and it can help lower your chances for future problems. The arteries will also have the elasticity that is needed to keep the heart strong, and it will reduce the chances by manifold.

Immune Booster

Your immune system is something you've got to take care of, and improving it can help. With running, you can improve your immune system greatly along with your cholesterol levels. In turn, you'll have a stronger body and less chances of getting sick.

Respiratory Heath

When you are running, your lungs will grow and expand/ contract in more dramatic ways to help get the breath that you need. You can improve your lung capacity, functionality, and even the use of them, and you can also help relieve symptoms of asthma to a degree if you run and build it up. It's a good way to help you get better, and if lung health is something you struggle with, then it's something of note that you should try out.

Running has a lot of benefits, and you'll be able to get the most of them when you do the activity. Do this, and you'll be a better runner than you'll ever be in no time.

Chapter 7: Tips to Make you the Best Runner You Can

Now that you know a lot about running, it's time to go over some tips to make you the best runner that you can be, and how to dramatically improve your running to be the best there is.

The first is to not strike with the heel of your foot. You should instead keep a more weightless stride to it. This can help to improve the chances of less back and knee pain.

Getting stronger is another major thing to do to help with your body. For some runners, there is a muscle imbalance that will make the body start to not work as well. Sometimes, runners have muscle weaknesses if they don't make sure to keep the rest of their body balanced and strong. Sometimes there is hip shifting which can cause other issues as well. What you should do is try to do some squats, planks, or even mild weight training, which we'll go over later on. This is a good tip that will allow you to improve your running efficiency and form over time.

Keeping a schedule is essential. You need to remember to go out to run whenever it's time to. Don't wait another moment once it is time. If you don't follow the schedule at the start, you won't get into the habit of running. Studies show it takes about 3 weeks for a habit to form for yourself, whether it is a personal rectifying of a bad habit, a good habit being put in, or whatever it might be. Running should almost be like a habit, and once it's time to run, do so. After a bit, it will be almost automatic for you to start, so you should do that.

Remember to keep your diet strong and keep at it. A good diet will improve your running abilities. If you're not eating well and running, you won't get better. Remember, your body is a machine in a sense, so you've got to fix the machine with the fuel necessary to have the best results possible. If you don't eat, you won't improve, and you won't get the confidence booster that you need.

When starting, do what makes you feel comfortable. Sure, you might be at the park and you see this woman running a lot faster than you are, but trying to match her pace can be trying on the body, and if you're not ready for it, it can lead to tiredness and injury. To start, run at your own pace, and when you're ready to increase it, do so for you. Remember, you're running for yourself, doing this to help benefit you, so you will need to make sure that you do keep your form going and you keep a pace that you can breathe in. You should ideally keep a pace where it's a bit of a challenge, but not so challenging that you are having trouble breathing. Do work for it, but if you want to, you can keep a talking pace that is right for you.

You should also make sure that you have sleep. A sleep-deprived body is one that will struggle on the runs, so it's best if you do make sure that you take the time to get sleep from time to time when you need it. In general, often we don't get nearly enough sleep that we need, so you should definitely make sure that you set an alarm, and do go to bed at the right time. Don't sit in front of the TV for hours upon hours after it's time to go to bed, and leave social media once you're ready to sleep.

Water is another major part of this, and for runners, you need to have enough water. A common problem many runners face when starting out is they don't drink enough water, and that is a surefire way to disaster. Water is necessary, and being dehydrated is a major problem. If you're dehydrated while running, it can be a struggle, and if you don't keep it in check, you could pass out, suffer from body issues, or even face other problems. One time, I didn't drink enough water before a longer run, and I nearly blacked out because I pushed myself too hard and I was dehydrated. You will want to make sure you drink at least 8-12 glasses a day, more so for the water you will lose from running.

For those who have a bit of sensitivity to temperature, it's best if you do take the time to choose a time of day that best fits you. If you don't want to run out in the direct sunlight and during the hottest parts of the day, run during the evening time or early morning, and avoid going out from about 10-3 because that is when it is hottest. If you can tolerate the heat, then by all means choose the time that fits you. I have sensitivity to the heat, and when it's too hot it can be hard to run, so I choose to run later in those instances. Remember, do what is best for you and if heat is your issue, do rectify that.

If you're struggling, get inspiration. There are many forums out there and even bodybuilding.com, livestrong.com, among many other fitness sites can be really helpful. Often, here are other users who are struggling to get in shape as well, and there are even running forums and sites that work best for you. You can create a little journal as well to track how you're feeling each day. In the end, you should do what is best for you, and you should make sure that you're keeping yourself going. If you need proper inspiration, you should get it, because the right inspiration can change everything, and it can make it even better for you, and often it can be the difference between running your best and not doing so hot at all.

Finally, get some support. If you have someone who is close to you and you feel would be a great running partner, get him or her involved. Remember, running isn't something only a few do. In fact, it's something that many can get into, many can accomplish, and many can achieve goals with. You have your own goals, but getting someone to work with you can make it even better for you. In general, the best thing to do in many cases is to be with someone who can help keep you going. If you struggle with maintaining a pace or a schedule, getting another involved and working with one another can be great. You might even pick someone slightly faster to give you a challenge after a while. Whatever it might be, get yourself going and running, and get the support that you need.

These tips will help you to become the best runner you can be. You should keep heed of these tips, use them when you can, and in general work to be the best you can be. Remember, you owe it to yourself to have a successful running experience, and if you do keep it successful and what's best for you, you'll end up having a much better time with this, and it'll be easier for you to handle over time.

Chapter 8: How to Prevent Running Injuries

Now, preventing running injury is just as important as maintaining a good pace and working towards bettering yourself. In truth, there are a lot of people out there who don't realize that the way they're running is a problem and it is causing strain on their body. This chapter will go over some of the things you can do to prevent running injuries.

The first is a general rule of thumb. If it hurts, don't push it. If you are in pain, take a day off. You should in general have one set day off for rest, maybe even two starting out. You need to have a rest day for your body to recover and build itself, and ideally, working up to running for about thirty minutes five days a week is the goal. You shouldn't push yourself if you are in pain, and if it hurts, don't make it worse.

Now, that's not to be confused with muscle soreness. If a muscle is sore, do go a bit easier on it to prevent further injury, but it is a natural thing that happens with any physical activity. You're working the boy out, improving the well-being of it, and in general you'll be able to have a better body after a little bit of soreness. If you're in pain, it should be better for you if you take a day off or a rest day, but soreness can be worked through.

If you do have sore muscles or strained muscles, you should ice them. Ice is good because it can help with the inflammation of the muscle. The cool heat and icy hot that some people use is also a good remedy, because often it will help make the injury way less, and in general it can work to improve your general health. If you do need to rest and ice something, do so because it is essential for the benefit of your life.

If you are struggling with going a distance and it's too much for you, don't make it worse if you can. You do want to try out newer and difficult tasks, but if it's risking an injury, don't do it. Work up to the ability that you can and once you feel ready, do go through with it. By the end of it, you will have a much better experience, and it will make things even better as well.

With anything, if you feel like there is something wrong, see a doctor. Sometimes, specialists can show you something you didn't even know about, and doctors can tell you if you're at risk for an injury. That's why it's imperative to go to the doctor and get a physical before starting, so you can watch out for things and get help when you need it. Knowing before you go can work to prevent injuries that are for sure.

Now, adding plyometric to the fray of a routing is really good, because it can help with muscle elasticity. It will help stretch it before a contraction, and because of this, it can help you improve you form and make it even better. Sometimes, skipping, leg bounding, or other plyo activities can be done beforehand to improve the elasticity of the muscles and to help it improve the stride that you have. Doing this can, also, help you to prevent injury.

Another major part of this is stretching. This is something most people will tend to forget, but it can mean big problems for you later on. You can do a bit of stretching beforehand, but you should make sure to do it after. This will prevent tightening muscles, strained muscles, and other such problems that can be a big issue with some people, and it does rectify the chances of injury for many people out there. If you feel like you might be at risk for straining something, take a bit more time to stretch before you go.

A slight warm up can help to improve the limberness of your muscles as well. Doing this will allow you to move better, faster, and have a better form. Sometimes, it also can help to warm up the muscles when it's cold, preventing them from getting strained while running. Even if it's just a simple warm up, it is best if you do take the time to get yourself going before you start running.

Shoes are also very important. It was said earlier in the book about the importance of them, but you should know that shoes could have a way of creating injuries in people. With the way the shoe molds to your foot and how it holds itself there, it can be a major issue for certain people if not taken care of. Often, people don't catch this until it's too late, when it starts to become a real issue for people. If you feel like you're not comfy in the shoes you're wearing, get some new ones. Always try them before you buy them, because while they might look pretty at first they can be a major problem with your feet over time. Prevent it from getting worse, and make sure you get the shoes that best fit you.

You should also stop landing on the midsole of your foot. If you land on your forefoot instead of on your heels, you will be able to have your weight of your body stabilized. This will also reduce the stress and impact that this could have on your joints, preventing further injuries as well. This is a good thing to have, and it will make it better for you as well.

Your stride is very important as well, not just for injury, but for your energy levels as well. If you leap forward and have a larger stride, you're prone to drained energy. What you will need to do is to stand tall and move your body a bit forward. When you feel like you're about to fall or have the falling sensation, then it's time to move forward just enough that you do catch yourself. If you keep that in mind and don't try to push it any more than that, you will have the proper stride. That way, it will take less energy, and it prevents muscle strain as well.

In the same vein, short strides are much better for you. A short stride will provide less wear on your body and prevent any possible injuries from happening. A shorter stride will make the movements in your joints less, such as in your knees, hips, and the ankles, and this win turn will prevent any straining or possible movement of the joints that should be happening. Start taking hurt strides, and help prolong the life of your body as well.

Now, we've said before that shoes shouldn't be uncomfortable, but they shouldn't be too comfortable either. The reason for that is that if you have the shoes being too supportive, it actually takes less strain off the rest of the body and the framework needed to support the foot. Now, and orthotic can help with the damage already there, and if your doctor says you need one, then get one. But, if your shoes feel so comfy that you're losing arch support, you will end up having problems because of it. It will make your foot weaker because of the lack of strain and strength on it, and this in turn can cause injuries to the shins, knees, and even the ankles. You should find a happy medium of comfort, but also an ability to keep the strength that you already do have in your feet and not letting them get weaker than they already are.

Now, you might want to run as hard as you can all the time. That might seem like a good idea on occasion when you want to push yourself, but if you do this all the time, injury is right around the corner. If you want to really get the efficiency you crave while running, you should instead do a slower speed and maintain a heart rate that is stable for yourself. If you do that, your body will have a much better result from this. You should train smarter, not harder. You can use a heart rate monitor to maintain the desired pace, and don't go past that set pace. This in turn will adapt the body to whatever the pace is that you want to be at, and in turn it will allow you to run comfortably around that pace. This is a great skill for those who want to run faster without going harder, and it will allow you to have a much better and more efficient body.

Preventing injury is important while running, and in truth, you should make sure that you do so. This chapter showed you some of the key things that you can do in order to prevent injury of your body and to help reduce the stress of the body. If you do this, it will improve your times over time, and you will become a much better runner as a result of these endeavors.

Chapter 9: Weight Training with Cardio

Finally, there is the question of weight training. Weight training is something that many people who start to run think about doing. Right now, since you are just starting out, you shouldn't worry so much about weight training, but this chapter will talk about the benefits, and some things that you can do.

The first thing is the benefits of this. Now weight training is very important for the body. In truth, many times runners who don't weight train end up hurting themselves. Weight training is something that you do need in order to improve one thing in the body that is essential: muscle strength. Runners who don't weight train suffer from weak joints, weak muscles, and it causes an imbalance, which can lead to injuries.

This doesn't mean you have to hit the gym and start to life weights 24/7. That's not the case with this. What you want to do, is balance out the muscle definition with the cardio, because to have the best body you can, you need both.

For some people, this can also help with the core. Your core is very important, because if you have an efficient one, you'll run well. It will also improve your stamina and strength as well, and coupling that with weight training can be great.

Some of the things you can do to help improve your strength are simple really. Planks, sit-ups, pushups, squats, and the like are good starts if you don't have equipment. Do some of these each day, and from there, work your way up in strength to weight training.

With weight training, you can get your own set of dumbbells, or even go to the gym. You should work on doing some bicep curls;

some practice with the strides to improve movement, and you should also work on improving your leg strength with squats. Using this with cardio will help you improve the strength of your body and make it better.

If you can, go to the gym. Memberships don't cost that much, and there is an array of equipment there. Weight training is important with cardio, and if you decide to be serious about running and go further, weight training is an element that will help you. Not only will it improve leg strength, it will help with your form too, which is very important.

Even if you don't want to start off with all of that, there is something small you can use to help you get started. Leg weights are little weights that attach to your legs. Use them while running to give you a bigger challenge. They can be a bit hard on your body at first but over time, you will have a much better experience from that, and soon, you'll be able to have an even better, stronger body, and you will be able to maintain a faster stride that works for you.

When you feel ready, incorporate weight training into your routines. It can be the best thing for you, and it can be something that will help you get much better over time, and it can make your dreams of being a better runner become a reality.

Conclusion

Thank you again for taking the time to check out this book!

I hope you learned all about running. This guide took you from the basic elements of what you will need to be the best runner you can be, to the other various parts of it that will help you. Running is a ton of fun, and there is a lot that you can do with it, and it's up to you to get the best results that you possibly can. You owe it to yourself to have a great body, have a great outlook on running, and doing it to help you become the strongest and best runner you can be.

With that in mind, there is the next step that you must take. This next step is simple, and that is to prepare yourself for running. Get the medical clearance, find clothing for you to run in, get a location squared away, and start putting a schedule together in order to start running. Running does take a bit of time and effort to do, and at first you might struggle with this. But don't fret about this don't worry, and instead work on this. You owe it to yourself to be the best runner you can be, and in truth, it can make your life all the more easier if you take it upon yourself to run, work on it, and have a stronger, healthier body than you ever expected to have before.